Cocoon of Love™
for Caregivers

ALSO BY SUSAN BROWNELL

Cocoon of Love™ for Cancer Caregivers
A beautiful read with a heart-warming
message of love for the caregiver

Cocoon of Love™ for Caregivers

Get Through the Tough Times
Surround Yourself with Love and Inspiration
When You Need It Most

Susan Brownell

Current Edition:
This book is the first in a series of books titled "Cocoon of Love™"

Copyright 2013 Susan Brownell

All rights reserved. No part of this book may be reproduced or utilized electronically without obtaining prior permission in writing from the Publisher.

DISCLAIMER:

This book is intended to offer inspirational support and encouragement for caregivers. It is not intended to provide medical advice or take the place of advice or treatment from trained medical professionals. If you have health questions or concerns about yourself or the loved one in your care, you should seek professional medical care. The publisher and author disclaim all liability that may be the result of the use of information contained within this book.

First Edition: October 2013

ISBN: 978-1-940826-01-1

Published by:
Susan Brownell
16124 Hardwood Road
Sparta, WI 54656
susanbrownell.com
sanctuaryforcancercaregivers.com

Printed in the United States of America
First Printing: October 2013

Dedication

To all caregivers, who give of themselves freely, as they care for loved ones, friends, neighbors, relatives, and patients in health care facilities. May your caring hearts and love be reflected back to you. May you inspire others to care with the compassion that only a caregiver knows.

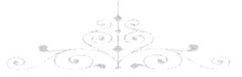

Contents

Introduction ix
1. Caregiver Attitude and Mindset 1
2. Grab onto Gratitude, Hope, Happiness, and Humor 25
3. Dealing with Worry, Change, and Fear 43
4. Living with Patience, Persistence, and Strength 61
5. The Art of Self-Care for Caregivers 85
6. Practicing Love, Compassion, and Kindness 103
7. Giving Care Through Faith, Comfort, and Courage 125
Acknowledgements 135
About the Author 137

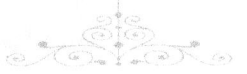

Introduction

The alarm clock is about to jump off the night-stand as you struggle to open your eyes so you can turn it off. You are exhausted. You feel physically and emotionally drained. Even so, you must go on. There's work, a school event, and a Doctor appointment for your aging mother. You don't want to look at the mountain of laundry rising up like a volcano from the ocean floor. You haven't even thought about what's for dinner tonight. You know you are just going to have to deal with all this, but some days it gets tough. It's tough to keep going physically. It's tough to stay in a positive mind-set. It's tough dealing with a loved one who is sick and depressed. It's tough to take care of yourself with all the daily demands.

This requires a lot of self-talk. What you need is the good kind. You need positive, realistic self-talk. Talk that lifts you up. Talk that encourages you. Talk that reminds you what you are made of. Talk that convinces you that you CAN do it. Finally, you need some talk to remind yourself to care for your most important "patient". That would be you—yes YOU! You need to continuously remind yourself that YOU are your most important resource to get through this caregiver journey. Whenever you purchase an important item, you need to take care of it so it will last a long time. The same is true of yourself. You need to protect yourself by practicing good eating habits, getting exercise, and enough sleep. You also need to have a little relaxation time to keep your spirits up.

How will you accomplish all of this? Your days are so full. You don't have much time to look for that much-needed inspiration to keep you in the right frame of mind. Caregivers need to continuously practice positive self-talk. Keeping your spirits up will help to keep your loved one's spirits up, as well. You need ongoing encouragement for your challenges and so that you can better deal with your loved one's challenges.

> *After several months of what was thought to be walking pneumonia, my mother had just been diagnosed with cancer. The Doctor's gave her six months. Then they said she had two months. She really had just two weeks.*
>
> *Things happened quickly. All seven of her children came home to be with her. Some traveled very long distances. As they sat with her, she felt the love. Time was quickly running out. One day she told my step-father, "I feel like I'm being wrapped up in a cocoon of love." What a wonderful gift for her children to give her!*

As you read this book, may you be encouraged an inspired. May you also experience a cocoon of love gently wrapped around you as you take the caregiver journey.

CHAPTER 1

Caregiver Attitude and Mindset

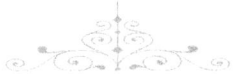

Attitudes are contagious. Is yours worth catching?

~ Unknown ~

Have you ever been around someone who is grumpy and a complainer? Did you notice after some time others started getting more negative too? The same is true of good attitudes. The positive, upbeat, and happy person at work is the one everyone likes and wants on their team. How's your loved one's attitude? If you display an encouraging, happy, and upbeat attitude, it will have a positive impact on their state of mind. If there's one thing you should want your loved one to catch right now, it's other people's good attitude.

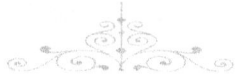

The most important opinion you have is the one you have of yourself, and the most significant things you say all day are those things you say to yourself.

~ **Unknown** ~

Self-talk is powerful. It will make you or break you. Use it wisely to get through challenging times. Instead of telling yourself you can't do it or it's too hard, try telling yourself you can do it. Talk to yourself about all the things you have done and all you have accomplished on this journey as a caregiver. Put notes around the house, in the car, and at work reminding yourself that you can do this. Make a tape of powerful self-talk affirmations of your self-worth, your strength, and the compassionate caregiver that you are. You are marvelous and don't you ever forget it!

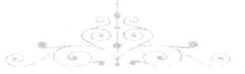

Forgive and forget.

~ English Proverb ~

Your loved one said some things to you that hurt. Perhaps he wasn't feeling well. Perhaps he was having a bad day and just angry in general at his situation. More than likely, he was just lashing out because of his frustration and anger over his illness. Do not take it personally. Let the words fade away. Don't dwell on it. Your loved one is going through a difficult time.

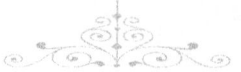

Death and life are in the power of the tongue, and those who love it will eat its fruit.

~ Proverbs 18:21 ~

Gossip. It's all around us. It is easy to participate in and difficult to refrain from. We have all given in to releasing some juicy tidbit of information at some point in our lives. It was so exciting at the time, but later the regret may set in and then it's too late. When a thought occurs, pause. Think before you say something. Do I know this to be true? Will my statement be hurtful to my loved one? Am I wording my information in a way that it can't be misinterpreted and create more havoc in someone's life? How many times have you said something only for it to be misunderstood and repeated in a less than desirable interpretation? When it comes to the loved ones we care for, we don't want to say anything to others that could accidentally be hurtful to them. Treat your tongue like a power tool to be handled with care. Be your own TV Censor. Put your tongue on a 5 second delay, so you can pause and self-edit.

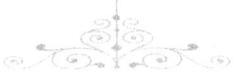

One of the healthiest habits you can have is to show forgiveness.

~ Susan Brownell ~

Forgiveness makes for a healthy giver and receiver. At times caregivers may be on the receiving end of some sharp comments. That can hurt. Sometimes caregivers are overlooked and not shown proper respect and appreciation by family members, friends, or the loved one they are caring for. On occasion, caregivers may even be wronged and lashed out at. Let go of the anger and resentment. Forgiveness is very cleansing and even in silence it sets a powerful example for others.

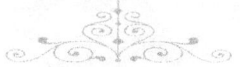

Whether you think you can or think you can't — you are right.

~ Henry Ford ~

You are a product of your thoughts. Make sure to play the positive mp3 music track and delete the negative mp3!

You've gotta dance like there's nobody watching,
Love like you'll never be hurt,
Sing like there's nobody listening,
And live like it's heaven on earth.

~ **William W. Purkey** ~

How do you keep that upbeat attitude when you are dealing with the serious things you are? You've heard it before. You have to live a good and happy life. You have to put yourself out there to live that good life. Yes, it's work. Yes, it takes effort. Give it all you've got to keep that upbeat attitude.

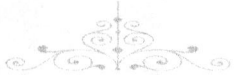

It is not doing the thing we like to do, but liking the thing we have to do, that makes life blessed.

~ Johann Wolfgang von Goethe ~

Most people would probably not choose to be a caregiver. It's tough work. When it involves a family member or friend it gets very emotional. It interferes with daily routines and social functions. Taking on the role of caregiver to a loved one is special. Because you love that person you care for, it makes it easier to like being their caregiver. Giving care to a loved one is a blessing. You may not see it that way at the time, but you will understand in time how blessed you were to be a caregiver.

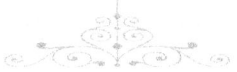

Life may not be the party we hoped for, but while we are here we might as well dance.

~ **Anonymous** ~

Life has a way of surprising us. It just doesn't always go according to our plans. Caregiving works the same. It may not be a party, but we deal with it as best we can. We look for every bit of enjoyment for our loved one and ourselves.

We might have to adjust our expectations of what will be a fun time. Suddenly we see life through a different perspective. What once may have seemed so insignificant and boring, may actually become something enjoyable and a future treasured memory. And so we dance. We may not dance as well as in the past. We may even dance with our partner in a wheel chair, but we do dance!

To live is the rarest thing in the world.
Most people exist, that is all.

~ Oscar Wilde ~

Do more than exist. Live, really live. Feel joy. Feel sorrow. Feel love. Be who you were meant to be. Don't hold back. Live your life. Yes, even as a caregiver, you can do that.

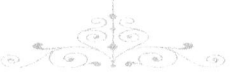

I am only one, but I am one. I cannot do everything, but I can do something. And I will not let what I cannot do interfere with what I can do.

~ **Edward Everett Hale** ~

You do a lot. You should not do it all. You do what you can within the confines of your circumstances. You accept that is the way it is. You may be one, but you are a great one!

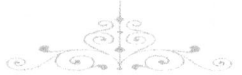

Believe you can and you're halfway there.

~ Theodore Roosevelt ~

When you've never done something before, you sometimes are scared. It is easy to convince yourself you can't do this and you can't do that. You don't know how and you are afraid of failure. Start telling yourself you CAN do this job of caregiving! You CAN work, care for your family and do your caregiving duties too. It may not be easy, but it can be done.

Get a dose of healthy inspiration. How? Join a support group. Read inspirational books. You can watch and study famous sports figures. There are plenty of them around who have overcome tremendous obstacles to their success. An amazing thing happens when you look at challenges others have overcome. Suddenly, our own obstacles seem smaller. They appear to be more doable than you first thought. Believe is a powerful word. You know you can do this. Just believe it and you'll be well on your way!

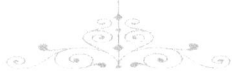

Write your sad times in sand.
Write your good times in stone.

~ **George Bernard Shaw** ~

So, your loved one is ill. You and your loved one may handle things in whatever way you choose. You can dwell on the sad, negative effects of the illness or you can remember the past good memories and try to create some new good memories. If you write your sad times in sand, the memories will fade like the tide gently washing away the sand. Sometimes it's good to forget. If you write your good times in stone, you will forever have them in your heart.

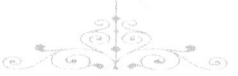

Life is short, live it.
Love is rare, grab it.
Anger is bad, dump it.
Fear is awful, face it.
Memories are sweet, cherish it.

~ **Unknown** ~

Too much of life is wasted not realizing it is slipping away. Caregivers see life with a clarity others don't. You must take what we have and make as many memories as you can. You must treasure times past and relive them with your loved ones. Sentimental memories mean a lot to loved ones who are ill. Help them preserve precious memories for others to remember in the future. It will mean a great deal to them now and to you in the future.

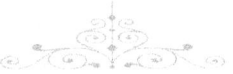

Things to Keep
Keep your thoughts positive,
because your thoughts become your words.
Keep your words positive,
because your words become your actions.
Keep your actions positive,
because your actions become your habits.
Keep your habits positive,
because your habits become your lifestyle.
Keep your lifestyle positive,
because your lifestyle becomes your destiny.

~ **Unknown** ~

Caregivers quickly learn that staying positive has a big impact on themselves and their loved one. Make a habit of being positive in all things. It will help conserve your energy and your sanity!

*All that we are is the result of what we have thought. The mind is everything.
What we think we become.*

~ **Buddha** ~

Tell yourself: I am a capable caregiver. Tell yourself: I can handle the physical care and the emotional care of my loved one. Tell yourself: I am getting better at this every day.

You know those things you've always wanted to do? You should go do them!

~ Unknown ~

As you see the impact of illness on your loved one, you experience your own sense of reality and mortality. If you have a Bucket List, look it over. What do you want to do? What do you hope to accomplish? What are your priorities? There are no guarantees in this life. Start to do some of those things. Live with no regrets.

"Nothing is impossible, the word itself says "I'm possible"!"

~ **Audrey Hepburn** ~

It can seem impossible—how do you find time to get it all done? Your loved one may feel recovery is impossible. Together the two of you can sit and commiserate about how impossible the situation is. Or, you can re-examine the word impossible. I'm possible? Is that for real? Yes! You can turn the impossible into the possible.

Choose a job you LOVE, and you will never have to work a day in your life.

~ **Confucius** ~

Do you think of caregiving as a "job" or a gift you give to your loved one? I love giving gifts, don't you?

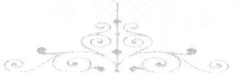

You must be the change you wish to see in the world.

~ Mahatma Gandhi ~

Much of the world news is very disturbing these days. You want the world to be a better place. You want people to share the values you have. In your own little corner of the world, you must set the example. You must show others how they should live their lives. In doing so, you are helping to make a positive change in the world for your loved one and for you.

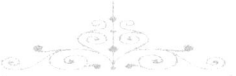

Write it on your heart that every day is the best day in the year.

~ Ralph Waldo Emerson ~

Did you know that positive self-talk has a tremendous impact on people? Caregivers need to strive for that self-cheer type of presence. Tell yourself each morning that it's a great day. Keep telling yourself that. Next, share that philosophy with your loved one. Say, "Good morning, Dad. It is a great day today. Not feeling so good? Well, we are going to see what we can do about that so we can make this one of the best days you've had for some time." How about "It's so beautiful outside," or "I just love cloudy days. It makes being in the house so cozy."

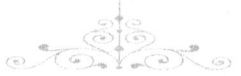

Do what you can, with what you have, where you are.

~ Theodore Roosevelt ~

Everyone's circumstances are different. Some caregivers live in with their loved one for 24-hour a day care. Some check in on their loved on daily. Some are long-distance caregivers orchestrating care from afar. Work within your means and within your circumstances. You may still have to work outside the home. You may have young children at home. You may have to travel with your job. Don't be too hard on yourself. Just do what you can and work on getting help with the remaining tasks. Remember, you are not Wonder-Woman or Super-Man!

CHAPTER 2

Grab onto Gratitude, Hope, Happiness, and Humor

Mix a little foolishness with your serious plans: it's lovely to be silly at the right moment.

~ **Horace** ~

You and your loved one both need some silliness in life! You just can't be serious all the time. Just a little silliness causes good feelings and relieves stress. Even in the course of serious illness, funny things just happen in daily life. Acknowledge them. Don't feel guilty about lightening things up a little. It's good for you and good for your loved one. Go ahead and laugh!

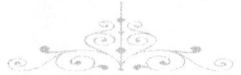

*Happiness is something to do,
something to love, something to hope for.*

~ Chinese Proverb ~

Caregivers definitely have something to do, something to love and something to hope for. Should they not also then have happiness?

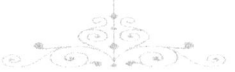

Things don't have to be perfect for you and your loved one to be happy.

~ Susan Brownell ~

It's strange how you change your perspective on life when illness strikes a loved one. Suddenly, it doesn't matter if you don't get that new car. It isn't that important if you get that promotion.

Caregivers redefine happiness. Your focus shifts to the little things. What can you make for supper that will be appealing enough to cause your loved one to eat? What can you do to ease their pain? How can you bring a bit of peace and comfort to them?

Suddenly you aren't so concerned about having the house clean and immaculate. You just want to savor time with your loved one and lift their spirits. It is no longer the end of the world if someone comes over and the house is not tidy. Instead of cleaning, you spent time looking at an old picture album and talking to our loved one. That brought a smile to their face and warmed your heart. It was worth a messy house to see your loved one's eyes twinkle as they spoke of years back.

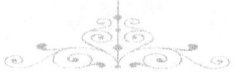

Those who wish to sing always find a song.

~ Swedish Proverb ~

Remember who you are as you go down the caregiver road. You still need to be you. Continue to do the things you love and be happy. It may not be quite the same, but don't lose yourself in this process. You owe it to your family. You owe it to yourself. It won't always be easy. If you make the effort, it will be worth it. Look for the good. Be positive. Enjoy your life to the best of your ability.

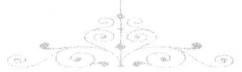

*He is a wise man who does not
grieve for the things which he has not,
but rejoices for those which he has.*

~ Epictetus ~

Gratitude is good for the soul! Caregivers have a lot to be thankful for. Even though the job is tough and the rewards are few, you can give thanks for any of the good little things that happen each day. Someone held the door open for you as you struggled with packages. Be thankful. A parking space opened up right next to the store. Be thankful. A neighbor offered to sit with your loved one while you attended a social event. Be thankful. Your loved one is ill. That weighs on you. Do not dwell on that, but rather look at the positive things happening every day in your life. Once you make an effort, you may be surprised to see just how many wonderful little things are happening in your life.

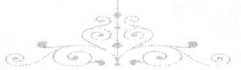

Each day is a gift. Don't send it back unopened.

~ Unknown ~

It's another day. Another day of work. Another day of caregiving. Another day of trips to the Doctor and pharmacy. Another day of trying to plan an appealing menu. Another day of trying to lift your loved one's spirits when you have all you can do to lift your own spirits. But…you have another day! Each day gives you another day together. Each day gives you another chance to comfort, love, and care for your special person. There are no returns and no exchanges on this day. Open the gift. Toss the ribbon and take the lid off the box. What will be in your gift today?

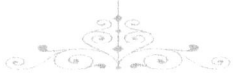

A good laugh and a long sleep are the two best cures for anything.

~ **Irish Proverb** ~

Sometimes you forget. You are a caregiver to someone with a serious illness. It is a somber time in both of your lives. Even so, you can still both laugh. Laughter is so cleansing. You will be quite surprised at all the things you can find to laugh about, even during your loved one's illness.

Your days are busy and it's difficult to get everything done. Sometimes you stay up late to accomplish it all. Don't deprive yourself of sleep. You will feel much better with a good night's sleep. Laugh first. Sleep last.

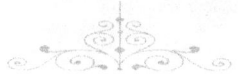

Joy is prayer - Joy is strength - Joy is love -
Joy is a net of love by which you can catch souls.
She gives most who gives with Joy.

~ **Mother Teresa** ~

Joy is a necessary component to a good life. Let down your net of love. Give from the heart with joy and start a joy revolution.

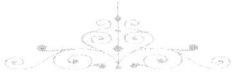

Face the sun, but turn your back to the storm.

~ African Proverb ~

There's nothing like the feel of the warm sun on your face after a long winter or summer storm. Turn your back on the bad that is behind you, and face the future with hope.

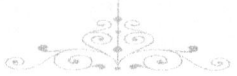

The most wasted day of all is that during which we have not laughed.

~ Nicolas Chamfort ~

The old saying of laughter being the best medicine has some merit. Try to find something each day to laugh about. It is so good for both the patient and the caregiver. It will lift your spirits, wash away some of the stress, and calm you. If you can laugh together, it can be a wonderful stress-reliever.

How do you find something to laugh at? Watch some comedies on television. Watch old family videos. Surf the internet for funny videos on YouTube and other sites. Watch "America's Funniest Videos" on television. Look for funny animal and children videos. There's an abundance of hilarious dog, cat, and baby videos. Read a joke book. Talk about funny things that happened over the years. Find something to laugh about every day. You don't have to be a comedian, just laugh!

A change is as good as a rest.

~ English Proverb ~

Caregiving can drain you. The days may be long and sometimes even depressing. Change it up a bit. Even if your loved one can't do all the things he used to, you can usually find something to break up the routine. It will make you both feel better. Take your loved one for a drive through some scenic country. Look at old pictures and reminisce. Put up a birdfeeder by the window and watch the birds.

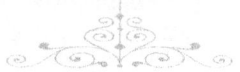

Count your blessings.

~ English Proverb ~

While focusing on someone with an illness, it is sometimes easy to lose sight of the good things in life. You have much to be grateful for. Start a gratitude journal and make entries every day. Some days you may have to look harder than others for something to be grateful for. Gratitude is a powerful force in one's life. Gratitude produces a healthy mindset to help get you through the tough times in life. What are you grateful for? Your loved one is grateful for you!

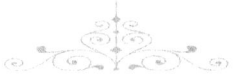

Life is a great big canvas, and you should throw all the paint on it you can.

~ **Danny Kaye**

If your life is a canvas, what would you want to leave behind on that canvas? Would you want lots of color and texture? Would you want lots of people? Would you want it to tell a story? Would you hold back and refrain from putting much on it? Would you want to only put on it fun things you want to do? Or would you want to share your canvas with your loved ones and friends?

Our days are all numbered. Your loved one knows that. Your loved one may or may not be able to do much, but they probably have certain things they hope to be able to do. Help them throw paint on their canvas while they can.

Now that you have helped your loved one paint their canvas, what will be on your canvas?

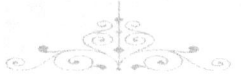

The secret of happiness is to count your blessings while others are adding up their troubles.

~ **William Penn** ~

Gratitude is the secret of a happy soul. We all have troubles. We all have various amounts of stress and unfortunate things happen in our lives. We can choose to dwell on that, or take a healthier approach.

We can also count our blessings. What are you grateful for? Did your loved one eat everything on his plate today? Did he sleep through the night? Is he feeling better?

Did you get to spend a little time reading your favorite new book? Did your daughter run some errands for you so you could rest? It may involve little things, but you probably have far more to be thankful for than you realize. Count your blessings instead of your troubles. Focus on positive, rather than negative. A positive mind is a powerful mind. A positive outlook yields a spirit of happiness.

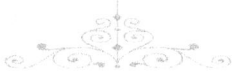

*Some endings are good.
They pave the way for new beginnings.*

~ Susan Brownell ~

As your loved one journeys through their illness there will be milestones. Perhaps it is the end of chemotherapy, a successful surgery, getting off a certain medication. Whatever the milestone, celebrate with your loved one. You have both been through this together. Be grateful for the milestones. Know that your lives which have been centered on this illness will continue to change—hopefully for the better! Make a cake. Fill a couple of balloons. Make a card for your loved one. Make their favorite dinner. Kick it up a notch by breaking out the good china and silverware. Make a toast—even if it's with apple juice!

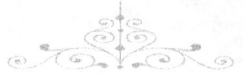

Happiness is when what you think, what you say, and what you do are in harmony.

~ **Mahatma Gandhi** ~

How do you define happiness? Your definition may vary at times, depending on what is happening in your life at the time. When all is well in life, happiness may be going on a wonderful vacation. When you are caring for a family member with a serious illness, happiness may be your loved one getting a good report from the Doctor.

CHAPTER 3

Dealing with Worry, Change, and Fear

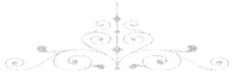

*Do not be anxious about anything,
but in everything, by prayer and petition,
with thanksgiving, present your requests to God.*

~ Philippians 4:6 ~

Instead of being worried and discouraged, you need to be praying. There are plenty of other things to take care of right now. Worrying is not on the list. Put in a red phone to heaven if you have to, but don't give up!

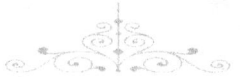

*Don't compromise yourself.
You are all you've got.*

~ Janis Joplin ~

In other words, don't overdo it! Far too many caregivers suffer from giving too much care for too long with little to no help. You are only one person. Get enough rest, eat right, exercise. Enlist the help of others so you can have a break sometimes. Preserve your own health.

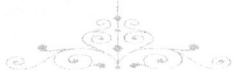

Do the thing you fear, and the death of fear is certain.

~ Ralph Waldo Emerson ~

Are you afraid to be a caregiver? That's understandable! It's scary for a non-medical professional to take on the responsibilities. There's no place you can be trained for 100% of the possible things you may have to deal with as a caregiver. You could sit and worry about it. You could enroll in some classes. But your loved one needs you now.

Just go ahead and start. You will learn as you go. Your confidence will increase and your fear will decrease. You are brave and caring to do what many others fear. You are facing your fear and doing it anyway. Did I tell you that you are awesome?

Do one thing every day that scares you.

~ Eleanor Roosevelt ~

Caregiving is scary. You don't know what will happen next, especially when dealing with a serious illness. As you face each of those challenges, your confidence will continue to increase. Caregiving develops character!

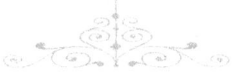

Far better it is to dare mighty things, to win glorious triumphs - even though checkered by failure - than to rank with those poor spirits who neither enjoy much nor suffer much, because they live in that gray twilight that knows neither victory nor defeat.

~ **Theodore Roosevelt** ~

Caregivers put themselves out there. Many go into the job not knowing exactly what they should be doing and build it from there. They know they can't wait to be a certified nursing assistant to start care-giving. They jump in immediately. They will make mistakes. They learn from them, minimize them, and move on in wisdom. They do what they have to do with no regrets. They enjoy the wins and don't dwell on the losses.

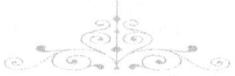

There are two things a person should never be angry at, what they can help, and what they cannot.

~ **Plato** ~

When illness strikes, anger often follows. Why did this happen to my loved one? You have no control over the fact that your loved one is ill. Anger will not change that.

How will I be able to be a caregiver and take care of all my other responsibilities? How will our lives change? What will we have to give up? These are things you will work through. Anger does nothing to change what you are dealing with.

Plato says we shouldn't be angry at things we can help and things we cannot help. That leaves us very little opportunity to be angry!

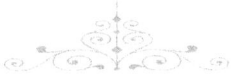

Never, never be afraid to do what's right, especially if the well-being of a person or animal is at stake.

~ **Martin Luther King Jr.** ~

Your loved one may be weak and vulnerable right now. There may be a question of physical safety and emotional well-being. Trust your gut. Do what you must to ensure they are safe. Even if they get angry, do what needs to be done to keep them safe and meet their basic needs.

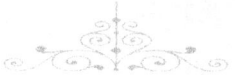

The best remedy for those who are afraid, lonely or unhappy is to go outside, somewhere where they can be quiet, alone with the heavens, nature and God. Because only then does one feel that all is as it should be.

~ Anne Frank ~

Our world is far too busy, too noisy and riddled with too much instant access to us via Social Media, Cell Phones and so forth. There is nothing like a walk in the woods when trials weigh on you. There is something very comforting about being alone with nature. Go for a walk. Sit and gaze at the beautiful landscape, the trees, the flowers, and the meandering river. Listen to the silence that we so rarely have a chance to experience anymore. Take some deep breaths and meditate on what is going on in your life and your loved one's life. Peace and calm will find you. Do these as often as you can. The more stressed you find yourself, the more often you should attempt to be alone with nature. If you are a religious person, this is a wonderful time to nurture your relationship with God.

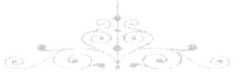

*Never bend your head. Hold it high.
Look the world straight in the eye.*

~ Helen Keller ~

You are following your calling. You are caring for a loved one in their time of need. Be proud and let the world know you answered the call. You are appreciated and needed. You are doing the right and honorable thing. You are someone's blessing!

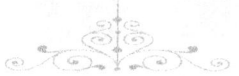

Life belongs to the living, and he who lives must be prepared for changes.

~ Johann Wolfgang von Goethe ~

Change is constant in the world of caregiving. Caregivers learn to adjust to change. They learn to be flexible. You wouldn't be doing this if you weren't ready to make changes as needed. Challenge yourself to problem-solve and make changes as needed. You are a genius!

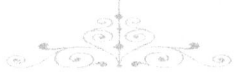

Life is either a daring adventure, or nothing.

~ Helen Keller ~

When it rains it pours as the old saying goes. Just when life seemed the busiest, you become a caregiver. Life can definitely become a daring adventure if you've never been a caregiver before. Even if you have been a caregiver before, it can keep you on your toes. You see, everyone responds a bit differently when they learn they have a serious illness or a life-changing disease. Some people may withdraw. Some may mourn the life they had previously. In that case, they may not want to go anywhere or do anything. Caregiving is an adventure. Are you up to the challenge?

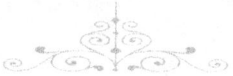

Who of you by worrying can add a single hour to his life? And if worry can't accomplish a little thing like that, what's the use of worrying over bigger things? Consider how the lilies grow. They do not labor or spin. Yet I tell you, not even Solomon in all his splendor was dressed like one of these. If that is how God clothes the grass of the field, which is here today, and tomorrow is thrown into the fire, how much more will he clothe you, O you of little faith!

~ **Luke 12:25-29** ~

We love to worry, don't we? We worry about our loved one's test results. We worry about people liking our new recipe. We worry about finances. God has told us not to worry, but we still do. God tells us to put our worries on him and have faith that he will handle all those things. That's one less thing for your To Do List. You no longer have to worry. Awesome!

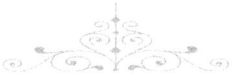

Worry is like a rocking chair. It gives you something to do, but gets you nowhere.

~ **Unknown** ~

Worry is a waste of energy. Caregivers need all the energy that they can get to deal with life. Practice energy conservation. Worry less and enjoy more free time and energy.

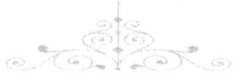

The glow of one warm thought is to me worth more than money.

~ **Thomas Jefferson** ~

In the midst of emotions and exhaustion, transport yourself away. Think of something you truly love to see or do. Think of someone who makes you feel wonderful. Think of a wonderful vacation or family event from the past. Think of some fun times you've had with your loved one. Think of something goofy or funny you did in the past. Think of the feel of a tight hug and a kiss. Wrap yourself up in the comfort of a cocoon—a cocoon of love.

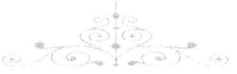

*It's not because things are difficult
that we do not dare; it is because we do not dare
that things are difficult.*

~ Seneca ~

Sometimes we make matters worse for ourselves because of our fears. Caregivers face this same dilemma. Because we are so afraid of what we might hear, we avoid open conversations with our loved one and their Doctor. In reality, open communication will lessen the stress. There will no longer be the opportunity to imagine the worse when we are as well informed as we can be.

CHAPTER 4

*Living with Patience,
Persistence, and Strength*

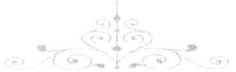

*If God sends us on strong paths,
we are provided strong shoes.*

~ Corrie ten Boom ~

Caregiving qualifies as a strong path. It's a tough, challenging trail. Go ahead, put on the strong shoes. You will be wearing them a lot as you hike the caregiver trail.

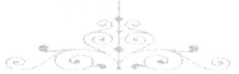

You have power over your mind - not outside events. Realize this, and you will find strength.

~ Marcus Aurelius ~

Are caregivers responsible for everything? Not really! You can control your thoughts, but not the test results, the surgery results, or the outcome of your loved one's illness. You can't control everything that upsets your loved one. As much as it may upset you, you can't even make your loved one eat. You need all the strength you can get to do what you must. Don't waste energy on things beyond your control. Put yourself in "Power-Saver" mode and save your strength for the things that really matter to you and your loved one. Remember, YOU have the power over your mind.

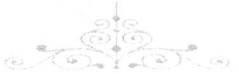

It is not fair to ask of others what you are not willing to do yourself.

~ **Eleanor Roosevelt** ~

As a caregiver, you will sometimes need to ask for help from others. Set the example by letting them see that you do some of the tasks you will be asking them to help with. Perhaps they feel uncomfortable about a task. You can gently guide them and show them what they need to know. Perhaps you could have them practice with your loved one before you leave. This will not only build their confidence, but also be reassuring to your loved one and you as well.

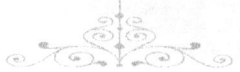

If we did all the things we are capable of, we would literally astound ourselves.

~ **Thomas Alva Edison** ~

Caregivers have a heavy schedule. How do you get it all done? There's the laundry, the shopping, the cleaning, the cooking, caring for your loved one. There are doctor appointments, pep-talks, and trips to the pharmacy. Getting organized and accepting help from others will help you streamline your To Do List. That's right. You can accomplish far more than you ever dreamed. Go ahead, amaze yourself!

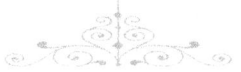

The first to apologize is the bravest.
The first to forgive is the strongest.
And the first to forget is the happiest.

~ **Unknown** ~

Sometimes caregiving can involve some tension. There can be tension with your loved one or tension with family members. Someone may say something they shouldn't have. Go ahead, apologize. But don't stop there. Don't let the poison get to you. Will this really matter a week from now? A year from now? Five years from now? Forgive, forget, and be happier.

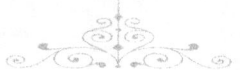

While we are postponing, life speeds by.

~ Seneca ~

Cancer Caregivers make life count! You do the tasks at hand, but you also remember there are many other things going on outside of the illness or handicap that you and your loved are dealing with. Time becomes even more precious to those struggling with their existence. Help them and yourself by trying to keep up a few of the family traditions. Celebrate holidays, birthdays, and decorate the house. It will cheer you both up.

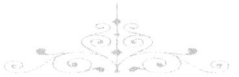

True strength is keeping everything together when everyone expects you to fall apart.

~ **Unknown** ~

As you slipped into your caregiver duties, you surprised yourself. Why not surprise them? You're finding that you CAN do this tough job. You ARE learning what it takes to help your loved one. You are getting more organized so that you may better handle the things coming at you. Others may be surprised to see the deep strength you have within you. They may be in awe. Go ahead; dazzle them at how together you are during this challenging time.

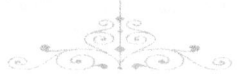

Little by little, a little becomes A LOT.

~ Tanzanian Proverb ~

No matter how good you are, you just can't do it all by yourself and not pay a price. Enlist the help of family, friends and social service agencies. It will help preserve your health and mental well-being. It will also help your loved one feel less of a burden to you. With many people helping it is not so much for one individual to deal with. Be the one to organize many helping hands. Each set of helping hands becomes a hug for you and your loved one. Who couldn't use a couple extra hugs during tough times?

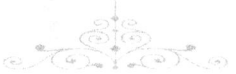

And we know that in all things God works for the good of those who love him, who have been called according to his purpose.

~ Romans 8:28 ~

We do not know why some things happen. We do know that God has a plan in all he does. We do know that he makes us stronger and wiser through all the challenges that come our way. He is always preparing us for the next thing. Learn what you can. Trust his promise. Something good will come from this. You don't know what will come from this or even when. There is one thing you do know for sure. Someday something good will come from this storm in your life. Learn what you can, so you will be ready when the good comes!

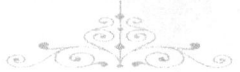

He who has not carried your burden does not know what it weighs.

~ Unknown ~

They have no idea what you are dealing with. They wonder why you can't go to the play with them next weekend. They don't understand why you are always so tired and busy. It is hard for you. Maybe it is time you told them just a bit about what you are dealing with. Those who have not been caregivers have difficulty realizing how demanding it is. If they knew your burden, they just might help you carry it!

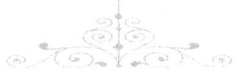

Courage doesn't always roar. Sometimes it is the quiet voice at the end of the night saying, "I will try again tomorrow".

~ **Unknown** ~

When things don't go as you'd like and you have doubts, be persistent. You can do this. You are learning. Your loved one is dealing with a tough thing in his life. You are brave enough to persist. You will keep trying, because you care.

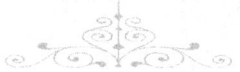

*One day, you'll be just a memory for some people.
Do your best to be a good one.*

~ **Unknown** ~

Although we like to think of caregiving as something we do for our loved one, we impact so many more lives. We are setting an example for our children, other relatives and friends in how to be compassionate and care for others. The impression we give them will touch their hearts. It will eventually cause other lives to be touched. It will keep the compassionate wheel of caregiving turning and moving along as others jump on the care-giver wagon.

You can't escape the responsibility of tomorrow by evading it today.

~ Abraham Lincoln ~

Plan and organize. Record lists of Doctors, Nurses, Friends, relatives, neighbors, phone numbers, addresses, medications, and pharmacies. Prepare and plan for various scenarios. Arrange for back-up help. Think about transportation, groceries, supplies, and medication refills. Make checklists. If something challenging happens, you will be ready and you will stress less.

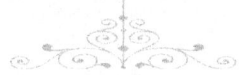

*I can do all things through him
who strengthens me.*

~ Philippians 4:13 ~

Caregivers of faith will not walk alone on their journey. They can turn to God to give them strength. They will be strong—Caregiver Strong!

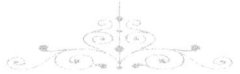

If you have no other choice, you'll be amazed at how much strength you can find within yourself.

~ Susan Brownell ~

You may be feeling some pressure right now. You have a lot going on in your own life and now you add to that being a caregiver. Your loved one may require a lot of one-on-one attention or may be seriously ill. This is when you reach down and draw on that inner-most reserve of strength. You know, the kind you think you don't have. The kind you have locked away in a vault and are saving for an emergency. There's no one else to do this job. If you don't, who will?

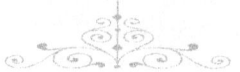

Don't be discouraged. It's often the last key in the bunch that opens the lock.

~ **Unknown** ~

There may be times when your loved one has shut down emotionally. He may not want to talk. He may be tired from the grueling treatments. He may be difficult to deal with at times. Hang in there and keep trying. Over time, you'll find what works to pull him out of his depressed mood. You'll get smarter and smarter about how to handle these challenging times.

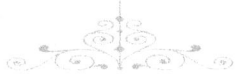

Take care of the minutes, and the hours will take care of themselves.

~ **Lord Chesterfield** ~

Avoid being overwhelmed. Focus on the little tasks that need to be done now. The minutes will fly by. They turn into hours as you care for your loved one.

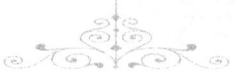

What lies behind us and what lies before us are tiny matters compared to what lies within us.

~ Ralph Waldo Emerson ~

It would be easy to focus on what your loved one has dealt with to this point. It would be easy to focus on what will come in the future for your loved one. What is most important right now is concentrating on what you can do to help the current situation. Focus on just one thing at a time to avoid getting overwhelmed.

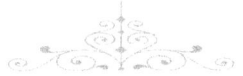

In three words I can sum up what I've learned about life: It goes on.

~ **Robert Frost** ~

How true this is! Your loved one may have a terminal illness. You have a lot to do to care for them. You also have a lot to do for your family. You must take care of yourself. You must eat right, get enough sleep and relax. Just because your loved one is seriously ill, it doesn't mean all the other things in your life have come to a stand-still. It is a constant in an ever-changing and turbulent world. Life goes on. Live it!

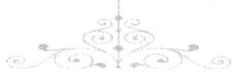

At the bottom of patience, one finds heaven.

~ West African Proverb ~

Patience. You want it. You need it. You seem to need a lot of it. You are forever practicing it. Keep on. This journey of patience will lead you to something very special. Just like you. Caregiver, you are special.

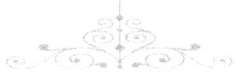

Start by doing what is necessary, then what is possible and suddenly you are doing the impossible.

~ **St. Francis of Assisi** ~

Caregiving can be overwhelming if you let it be. Just like any task that feels like it's too much, you need to chunk it down. Decide what the priorities are at this time. Is it most important to make the living arrangement safer? Does your loved one need assistance in keeping track of medications? Is pain control the priority? Is transportation to and from treatments needed? Just focus on what's urgent right now. Get that under control first. Next, start working on the lower priority items. Over time you will get a routine going. Before you know it, you will be doing so much more than you thought you could when you were trying to do it all at once.

CHAPTER 5

The Art of Self-Care for Caregivers

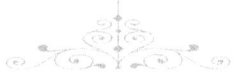

You give but little when you give of your possessions. It is when you give of yourself that you truly give.

~ **Kahlil Gibran** ~

Caregivers are givers. You give care, you give food, and you give little gifts. You give transportation. You give a shoulder to cry on. You give a listening ear. You give encouragement. You give from your heart. You give your love. You give yourself. In doing so, you give what no one else can. No one else can give that loved one the same thing you can—the same love, the same encouragement, or the same hope in the way that you do. Perhaps that is why it is you that is caring for them instead of someone else.

Give of yourself to them, but also give of yourself to you. Protect your health. Get as much rest as you can. Eat nutritious meals and get exercise. This will not be easy. As a caregiver you tend to focus on them. Don't forget the most important person you give care to is yourself!

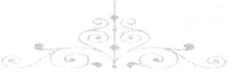

*One cannot think well, love well, sleep well,
if one has not dined well.*

~ Unknown ~

How can you care for them if you don't care for yourself? In all the activities of giving care and your own daily life, how often have you skipped a meal or not eaten right? It's simple, but important. Care for yourself to maintain your health and well-being. That way, you can be there for them!

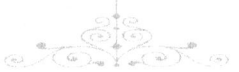

Remember always that you have not only the right to be an individual, you have an obligation to be one.

~ **Eleanor Roosevelt** ~

So you are a caregiver. That is true. But you are so much more than that. You are a kind, giving, and compassionate person. You are a person who has friends and family who love having you in their lives. You are a person who has hobbies and perhaps a job outside the home. You are a person like none other. Don't lose yourself as a caregiver. Make every effort to maintain who you are. Don't give up everything to give care to your loved one. You owe it to yourself to take care of you too!

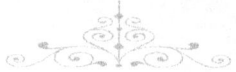

I cannot trust a man to control others who cannot control himself.

~ **Robert E. Lee** ~

You have a big responsibility. Watch their medicines. Make sure they get to their appointments. Make sure they eat right. Watch for new symptoms.

You are actually a caregiver to two. You care for your loved one and yourself. It takes discipline to keep oneself under control and not overdo it when caring for another. Remember that if you are burned out, you won't be much help in caring for your loved one. Just as in an airline emergency, you should always put the oxygen mask on yourself first, then help your fellow passengers.

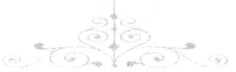

*Early to bed and early to rise,
makes a man healthy, wealthy and wise.*

~ **English Proverb** ~

When caring for others, you may tend to neglect yourself. Be mindful of the need for self-care. Get as much sleep as you can. Eat healthy. Try to get a little exercise. As a caregiver, your number one patient should be you!

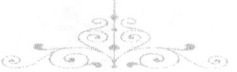

A light heart lives long.

~ Irish Proverb ~

Preserve your health! Keep it light. No long face. No doom and gloom. Deflate the stress balloon to make it light. Less pressure lightens the load.

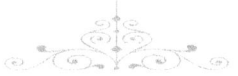

For God gave us a spirit not of fear but of power and love and self-control.

~ 2 Timothy 1:7 ~

God will help caregivers overcome the fear. Through his love, you receive strength to accomplish the tasks set before you. He helps you control your emotions at a time when they are tested. He will also tell you when you are operating at maximum capacity. Listen to your instincts. Your God-given spirit will see you through. Trust this is true and feel a great sense of relief!

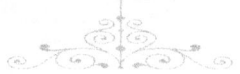

Never worry about numbers. Help one person at a time, and always start with the person nearest you.

~ Mother Teresa ~

Do you ever feel like everyone needs something from you? Do you feel like it's too much and you just can't do it all? Focus on the priorities. Who needs your help the most? Help them. Teach others what they can do to help themselves and each other to lessen their dependence on you.

You do not have to do it all. Communicate what you are dealing with to your family. It's not a competition to see who has helped the most people. It's about taking care of who needs help the most. And remember to include yourself in the mix. You need to help yourself too. You won't be much help to others if you are exhausted and sick from overdoing it. Slow down…there are more days in the week!

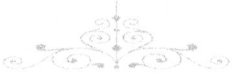

Every day we should hear at least one little song, read one good poem, see one exquisite picture, and, if possible, speak a few sensible words.

~ Johann Wolfgang von Goethe ~

Caregivers can get immersed in daily living and the long To Do List. They must get in the habit to ensure they reserve some time each day for a little get-away time. This may be for only a few minutes at a time, but it is so important to well-being. Music lifts the spirit. Reading is therapeutic. Visual images can create a kaleidoscope of happy thoughts. Having a conversation with someone about something other than caregiving provides a release from the continuous exposure to caregiver tasks.

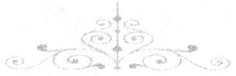

You yourself, as much as anybody in the entire universe deserve your love and affection.

~ **Buddha** ~

How much do you do for your loved one? How much do you love them? Do you love yourself just as much? Treat yourself to something. Take a break. Read, take a walk, watch the birds, and pet the dog or cat. You would do it for them, so why not do it for yourself? Think of your best qualities. You are awesome. Celebrate your greatness!

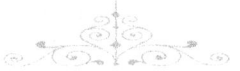

You are what you eat.

~ English Proverb ~

You know it's true. You've heard it for years. Eat right and avoid too much fast food and processed food. You will feel better and protect your health. You are a caregiver. You are under stress. You need to feel good!

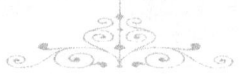

Life is really simple, but we insist on making it complicated.

~ Confucius ~

Caregivers have a lot on their plate. It doesn't have to be complicated. It may be a lot to do and deal with, but focus on what's most important. Just do what you have to do. Consolidate trips to save extra driving around. Organize shopping lists. Take shortcuts when possible, and get help!

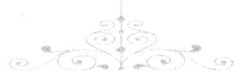

*Carve out some alone time for yourself.
You need to care for yourself too!*

~ **Susan Brownell** ~

Give yourself a gift that only you can give—some time alone. Do whatever you want. Read a book or go in another room and shut the door while you watch a favorite television show. Do some crafts. Practice your hobby. Meditate. Exercise. What invigorates you? What relaxes you? What is something you really look forward to? Make your family and friends aware that this is your time and that you don't want to be disturbed.

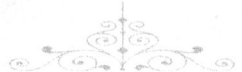

*I am thankful to all those who said no,
it's because of them I did it myself.*

~ Albert Einstein ~

Don't resent those who refused to do the caregiving job you are doing. Rejoice that you are getting an experience to be closer to your loved one and know them in a way you never would have otherwise. Your life will never be the same after this experience. You will be a better, kinder, more compassionate person. You will be blessed!

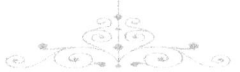

Fear less, hope more, eat less, chew more, whine less, breathe more, talk less, say more, love more, and all good things will be yours.

~ Swedish Proverb ~

This is how caregivers live their lives—more or less! Because of that lifestyle, all good things are heading your way!

CHAPTER 6

Practicing Love, Compassion, and Kindness

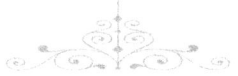

Kind words will unlock an iron door.

~ Turkish Proverb ~

Sometimes you feel like you are getting nowhere. Sometimes a loved one who is ill just puts up a wall and locks the door. They may not want to talk. They are grieving their changed life. They may be bitter and resentful. They may be sad and depressed. Respect their need for some alone time. Don't take their actions personally. Speak to them with kindness and eventually most will eventually come back to you.

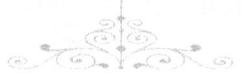

He who loves you, loves you with your dirt.

~ African Proverb ~

Love is unconditional. We all have some dirt. If we really love someone, we love them unconditionally, dirt and all. Caregivers get to see people's dirt more than most people. Caregivers love them no matter how much dirt they have.

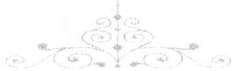

Love is the beauty of the soul
~ Thomas Edison ~

Caregiver, as beautiful as your soul is, you must have a lot of love.

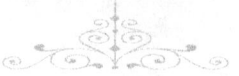

Be kind whenever possible. It is always possible.

~ Dalai Lama ~

Some days our loved one may not be at their best. They may be grumpy. They may not want to take their meds or a bath. They may complain about the food. They may even insult you, the one who does so much for them. Wear your caregiver suit of armor and let the comments ricochet off like they never said those hurtful things.

Your loved one may not be feeling well. They may be mourning the life they used to have. They may be worried about what their future holds. They may be worried about some upcoming medical tests or test results. They may resent that someone has to do all these things for them. They may be angry that someone has to take care of them.

Try to be kind and understanding. Know that they are not themselves right now and really don't intend to hurt you.

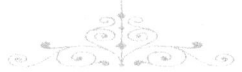

Home is where the heart is.

~ English Proverb ~

People who are sick generally prefer to be home. If you have the proper accommodations and are able to do the necessary tasks, try to work with your loved one on this. If you can't do this, see about getting volunteers or hiring someone. It will help your loved one to feel some semblance of life being normal if they can be at home and if you can handle it. If you can't do it (and not everyone can) don't beat yourself up over it. Think about ways to bring a little bit of home to your loved one when you visit him at his new location. Bring photos, favorite knick knacks, a favorite chair or anything special to your loved one. Home really is where the heart is and your heart is with him.

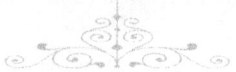

Kindness is a language which the blind can see and the deaf can hear.

~ **African Proverb** ~

The language of kindness has no letters or sounds. It is love and actions. The dialect of kindness may vary slightly, but it is in essence, a hug from the heart of one to another. The language of kindness is the earth's one universal language. Caregiver, you speak the language fluently!

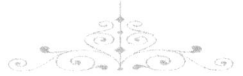

Love comforteth like sunshine after rain.

~ **William Shakespeare** ~

Sometimes there's not much you can do. If the Doctor has bad news, all you can do is be there. Your loved one will feel your love in the touch of your hand and the gaze of your eyes.

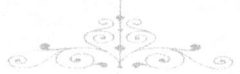

Be kind, for everyone you meet is fighting a hard battle.

~ Plato ~

Your loved one is facing challenging times. There's the physical illness and the mental battle as well. There's not feeling well physically and there's sadness at a new kind of dependency on others. As the internal conflict occurs within your loved one, sometimes they may lash out at others. Understand this is all normal and your loved one doesn't really want to hurt you. Instead of responding in a like way, pause, take a deep breath, and respond with kindness. The war they are waging is real and it is difficult. Be kind.

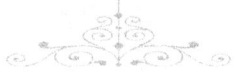

Many hands make light work.

~ English Proverb ~

Get others to help you. You don't need to do this alone. Ask friends, neighbors, and relatives to pitch in. Every little bit helps. Let them know when you are overwhelmed. Sometimes others assume you have everything under control, so they don't offer. Many people are willing to help if you just let them know.

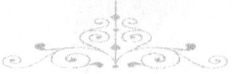

Silence is golden.
~ English Proverb ~

Your loved one isn't talking much. That doesn't mean they aren't thinking. You are thinking too. Sometimes there are too many questions and too many reminders of the current health situation. Sometimes silence is the best coping mechanism. Just because your loved one isn't talking to you, it doesn't necessarily mean he's angry at you. It's okay. You can talk another time. Silence is sometimes a "get-away".

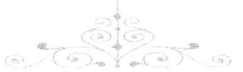

He who shines, will let the light fall on those next to him.

~ Unknown ~

Caregiver, you are much more of an inspiration to your loved one than you will ever know. Shine your light on your loved one and let him bask in its glow. Maybe, just maybe, some of it will be reflected back to you.

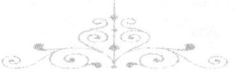

Love is a bridge between two hearts.

~ English Proverb ~

Caregivers truly know the meaning of love. They live love daily. Here's to building bridges!

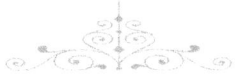

No three words have greater power than I Love You.

~ Unknown ~

So true! Don't be shy. Go ahead. Say it. Tell your loved one that you love them. Too often we don't say it when we should. Live with no regrets. It's simple. "I love you!" That wasn't so hard, was it?

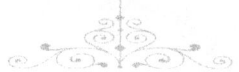

*The most I can do for my friend
is simply be his friend.*

~ **Henry David** ~

What a wonderful gift it is to be a friend. It's like a two-way gift. The giver and the receiver both receive a something. Sometimes the best gifts are free, unwrapped and priceless. Be a friend to the one you care for. He needs all the friends he can get right now.

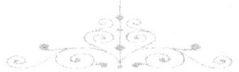

Friends are those rare people who ask how you are and then wait to hear the answer.

~ **Unknown** ~

Friends care. They want the best for you. They hurt with you and celebrate with you. Friends are like family, and sometimes better than family. Good friends really listen. Good friends don't have an agenda. Caregivers are friends in every sense of the word.

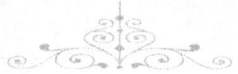

A friend loves at all times, and a brother is born for adversity.

~ Proverbs 17:17 ~

Sometimes your loved one may not be so easy to love! They may be going through a rough day. Remind yourself they are not quite themselves. Remind yourself how tired and stressed your loved one is. Remind yourself to not take this personally.

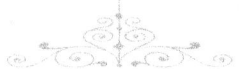

To the world you may be one person, but to one person you may be the world.

~ **Unknown** ~

Sometimes you may feel you can't possibly do it all. You may even tell yourself, "I am only ONE person! I can't do all this." Save some of yourself to spend some time with your loved one, even on the busy days. You are their North Star. They need you and want you in their life. You are the world to them.

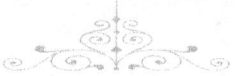

The dew of compassion is a tear.

~ Lord Byron ~

You are compassionate. You wouldn't be a caregiver if you weren't. Because you care, it sometimes hurts. You start to tear up. You don't have to turn your face away. Your loved one sometimes needs to see your raw emotion to know how much you care. It's okay to cry sometimes.

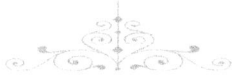

When an old man dies,
a library burns to the ground.

~ African Proverb ~

Your loved one has much to share. Now is the time to learn about his past. Now is the time to share the heritage, the history, the fun, pranks, hard work, and ancestry of him. Now that he is ill, you will see a side you've never seen before. He will love telling the old stories. He will light up when talking about his history. Show an interest. Fire up his neurons to relive the memory of his youth. Now is the time to learn what he has written on the pages of his life.

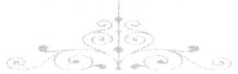

Every time you SMILE at someone, it is an action of love, a gift to that person, a beautiful thing.

~ **Mother Teresa** ~

Sometimes words fail us. Sometimes we are so close to the situation. It is then we practice non-verbal communication. Is your loved one having a rough day? Look in their eyes. Flash a smile at them. Touch their shoulder or hand. They will feel your love. They will be lifted up. They may not show it, but they will be affected.

CHAPTER 7

Giving Care Through Faith, Comfort, and Courage

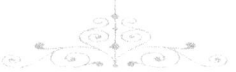

You can never cross the ocean until you have the courage to lose sight of the shore.

~ **Christopher Columbus** ~

Caregiving is scary. Fear is a challenging thing to overcome. Facing your fear and gaining courage makes one stronger and better able to accomplish the things you need to do. Every day is an unknown. Medical drama can prevail, although most caregivers hope that will be minimal. Emotional drama takes a toll also. If you didn't have the courage to shove the boat off from the shore, you would not be as effective. Trust your compass and sail on. You will be just fine!

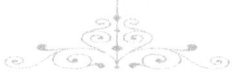

Better a dry crust with peace and quiet than a house full of feasting, with strife.

~ Proverbs 17:1 ~

If your loved one has a friend or relative that you find upsets him greatly, it may be better for that individual to stay away. Sometimes when people are ill, they don't care to interact with certain people. Sometimes your loved one can appear to be grumpy or rude. If your loved one is seriously ill, and upset by someone's presence, you may need to intercept the visitor in your own tactful way.

*In his heart a man plans his course,
but the LORD determines his steps.*

~ Proverbs 16:9 ~

Turn it over to the Lord. He will help lead you down the correct path.

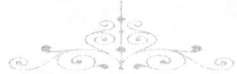

The best way to gain self-confidence is to do what you are afraid to do.

~ **Unknown** ~

When it comes time to be a caregiver, don't just sit there! Jump right in. You'll learn as you go. It is sink or swim and you are going to swim! Start with baby steps. Take advantage of the resources available to help caregivers. Take a caregiver class. Research the internet. You'll learn. No one has all the answers starting out. The more you do, the better you'll get at this. The better you get, the more your confidence will grow. You did it. You were afraid, but you did it anyway. You are amazing!

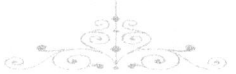

Faith will move mountains

~ English Proverb ~

If you are a person of faith, lean on it. If your loved one is a person of faith, encourage them. If your loved one is not a person of faith, they may desire to learn more about religion at this time in their lives, but not know who to talk to or how to go about it. Help them find some inspirational religious shows on TV. Offer to take them to a local church. Most churches offer a shut-in program with home visits. Some churches have a Family Minister specially trained to help individuals deal with illness and matters of faith. Faith helps when facing illness.

Let God's promises shine on your problems.

~ Corrie Ten Boom ~

God will never send more to you than you can endure. Put all your burdens on him. Feel yourself get lighter. What a relief to not have to carry the burdens! Talk to him as if he were your best friend because he is. Tell him all you and your loved one are enduring. Ask for his help. Believe he will answer your prayers. Wait, watch, and listen. Be amazed at what happens in big and little ways all around you!

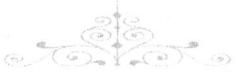

We learn something from everyone who passes through our lives. Some lessons are painful, some are painless. But, all are priceless.

~ **Unknown** ~

Caregivers experience things that others won't. They learn medical procedures and warning signs. They learn about the emotional impact of illness on their loved one and the family. They learn about resilience and determination. They see the human spirit at a time of great challenge. Just as you touch them at this difficult time, they leave an impression on you. Caregivers learn about life. Sometimes it takes courage to learn priceless lessons in life's classroom. Sometimes it hurts. Sometimes it is a very personal, priceless gift.

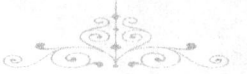

You will never do anything in this world without courage. It is the greatest quality of the mind next to honor.

~ Aristotle ~

Caregiver, you have the wonderful quality of courage. You have taken on a job many fear. You do what must be done for your loved one. You learn as you go and are an example for others. Feel good about what you do. You are respected and loved for what you do. Your loved one may not say it, but each time your eyes meet, a big "Thank You" scrolls across his face. Although he may never say it, he is thinking, "Thank you. Thank you for your courage to help me face my challenges. Thank you for your courage to do what others can't or won't. Thank you for taking precious time from your life to make mine better. Thank you for your love and compassion. Thank you for caring for me in my time of need."

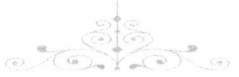

Acknowledgements

Cover Illustration by: Dima Krasovski
Cover Illustration rights belong to the author.

With thanks to some special people in my life:

> My husband for his support, my children and grandchildren who endured my absence as I wrote.
>
> My parents and mother-in-law, who through their illnesses and aging taught me what is at the heart of caregiving.

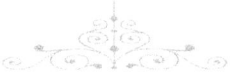

About the Author

Susan Brownell is the Founder of SanctuaryForCancerCaregivers.com website. Over a consecutive eight-year period her mother, father, step-mother, and step-father were diagnosed with cancer. One by one they were diagnosed. One by one they left this earth. Susan has also helped care for other aging and sick relatives.

Susan struggled with the stress and exhaustion of caregiving. She knows the pain and the heartbreak. She knows the physical and emotional toll caregiving takes. Susan believes every caregiver could use a healthy dose of encouragement and inspiration to get them through the tough times.

Susan has authored another book in the "Cocoon of Love" series. It is called, "Cocoon of Love for Cancer Caregivers: Get Through the Tough Times, Surround Your Loved One and Yourself with Love When You Need It Most"

Besides writing, one of Susan's passions is to help caregivers with their daily struggles. She wishes she would have had some help available when she was starting her role as a caregiver. Watch her websites for information on upcoming books and teleseminars to help caregivers.

To keep up with the latest from Susan visit:
sanctuaryforcancercaregivers.com
susanbrownell.com

www.ingramcontent.com/pod-product-compliance
Lightning Source LLC
Chambersburg PA
CBHW031359040426
42444CB00005B/345